This Planner Belongs To:

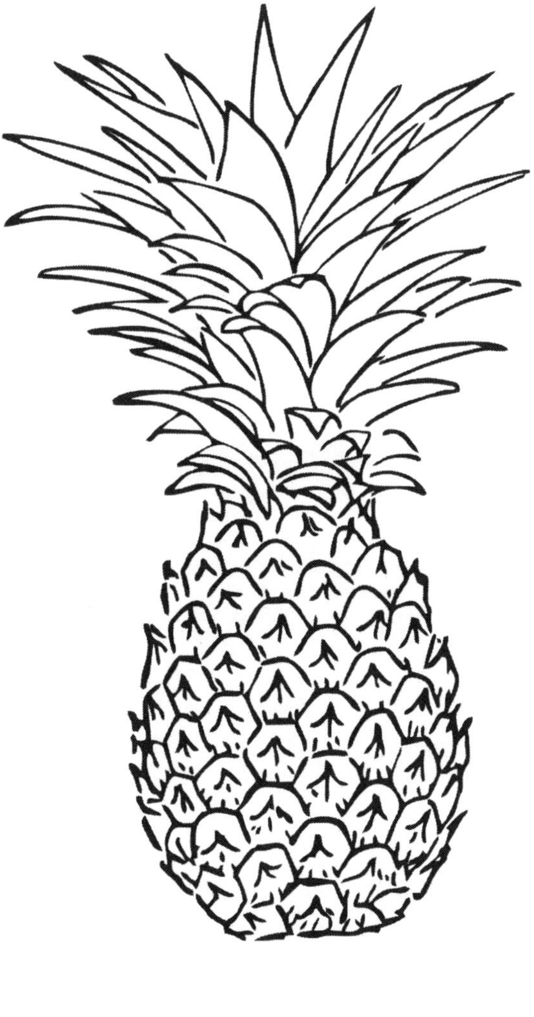

Cycle Tracker

Month:___________

Sunday	Monday	Tuesday	Wednesday	Thursday	Friday	Saturday

Cycle Tracker

Month:___________

Sunday	Monday	Tuesday	Wednesday	Thursday	Friday	Saturday

Cycle Tracker

Month:___________

Sunday	Monday	Tuesday	Wednesday	Thursday	Friday	Saturday

Cycle Tracker

Month:____________

Sunday	Monday	Tuesday	Wednesday	Thursday	Friday	Saturday

Cycle Tracker

Month:________________

Sunday	Monday	Tuesday	Wednesday	Thursday	Friday	Saturday

Cycle Tracker

Month:__________

Sunday	Monday	Tuesday	Wednesday	Thursday	Friday	Saturday

Cycle Tracker

Month:__________

Sunday	Monday	Tuesday	Wednesday	Thursday	Friday	Saturday

Cycle Tracker

Month:__________

Sunday	Monday	Tuesday	Wednesday	Thursday	Friday	Saturday

Cycle Tracker

Month:___________

Sunday	Monday	Tuesday	Wednesday	Thursday	Friday	Saturday

Cycle Tracker

Month:__________

Sunday	Monday	Tuesday	Wednesday	Thursday	Friday	Saturday

Cycle Tracker

Month:___________

Sunday	Monday	Tuesday	Wednesday	Thursday	Friday	Saturday

Cycle Tracker

Month: ____________

Sunday	Monday	Tuesday	Wednesday	Thursday	Friday	Saturday

Appointments

Date	Time	Doctor	Questions	Notes

Appointments

Date	Time	Doctor	Questions	Notes

Retrieval Medications

Medication	Dose																															

Medication	Dose																															

NOTES & REMINDERS

Retrieval Results

Retrieved	
Fertilized	
Day 3	
Day 5	
Made to freeze!	

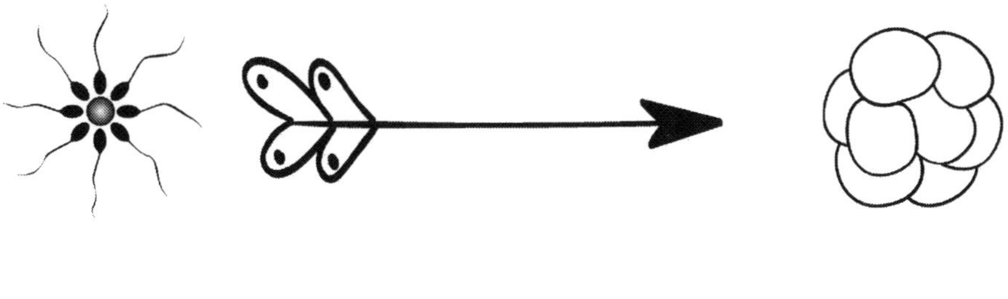

Transfer Medications

Medication	Dose																															

Medication	Dose																															

NOTES & REMINDERS

My Week at a Glance

Week of: ____________________

MY WEEKLY AGENDA: NOTES

Sunday..

Monday..

Tuesday..

Wednesday..

Thursday..

Friday..

Saturday..

TOP GOALS

TOP TO DO OF THE WEEK

HEALTHY EATING TRACKER

M	T	W	T	F	S	S

QUOTE OF THE DAY

TODAY I AM GRATEFUL FOR:

My Week at a Glance

Week of: ____________________

MY WEEKLY AGENDA: NOTES

Sunday..

Monday..

Tuesday..

Wednesday..

Thursday..

Friday..

Saturday..

TOP GOALS

TOP TO DO OF THE WEEK

HEALTHY EATING TRACKER

M	T	W	T	F	S	S
☐	☐	☐	☐	☐	☐	☐
☐	☐	☐	☐	☐	☐	☐
☐	☐	☐	☐	☐	☐	☐
☐	☐	☐	☐	☐	☐	☐
☐	☐	☐	☐	☐	☐	☐
☐	☐	☐	☐	☐	☐	☐
☐	☐	☐	☐	☐	☐	☐
☐	☐	☐	☐	☐	☐	☐

QUOTE OF THE DAY

TODAY I AM GRATEFUL FOR:

My Week at a Glance

Week of: ____________________

MY WEEKLY AGENDA: NOTES

Sunday..

Monday..

Tuesday..

Wednesday..

Thursday..

Friday..

Saturday..

TOP GOALS

HEALTHY EATING TRACKER

M	T	W	T	F	S	S
☐	☐	☐	☐	☐	☐	☐
☐	☐	☐	☐	☐	☐	☐
☐	☐	☐	☐	☐	☐	☐
☐	☐	☐	☐	☐	☐	☐
☐	☐	☐	☐	☐	☐	☐
☐	☐	☐	☐	☐	☐	☐
☐	☐	☐	☐	☐	☐	☐
☐	☐	☐	☐	☐	☐	☐

TOP TO DO OF THE WEEK

QUOTE OF THE DAY

TODAY I AM GRATEFUL FOR:

My Week at a Glance

Week of: ____________________

MY WEEKLY AGENDA: NOTES

Sunday..

Monday..

Tuesday..

Wednesday..

Thursday..

Friday..

Saturday..

TOP GOALS

HEALTHY EATING TRACKER

M	T	W	T	F	S	S
☐	☐	☐	☐	☐	☐	☐
☐	☐	☐	☐	☐	☐	☐
☐	☐	☐	☐	☐	☐	☐
☐	☐	☐	☐	☐	☐	☐
☐	☐	☐	☐	☐	☐	☐
☐	☐	☐	☐	☐	☐	☐
☐	☐	☐	☐	☐	☐	☐
☐	☐	☐	☐	☐	☐	☐

TOP TO DO OF THE WEEK

☐ ____________________

☐ ____________________

☐ ____________________

☐ ____________________

QUOTE OF THE DAY

TODAY I AM GRATEFUL FOR:

My Week at a Glance

Week of: ____________________

MY WEEKLY AGENDA: NOTES

Sunday...

Monday...

Tuesday...

Wednesday...

Thursday...

Friday...

Saturday...

TOP GOALS

HEALTHY EATING TRACKER

M	T	W	T	F	S	S
☐	☐	☐	☐	☐	☐	☐
☐	☐	☐	☐	☐	☐	☐
☐	☐	☐	☐	☐	☐	☐
☐	☐	☐	☐	☐	☐	☐
☐	☐	☐	☐	☐	☐	☐
☐	☐	☐	☐	☐	☐	☐
☐	☐	☐	☐	☐	☐	☐
☐	☐	☐	☐	☐	☐	☐

TOP TO DO OF THE WEEK

QUOTE OF THE DAY

TODAY I AM GRATEFUL FOR:

My Week at a Glance

Week of: ____________________

MY WEEKLY AGENDA: NOTES
Sunday......................................
Monday......................................
Tuesday......................................
Wednesday......................................
Thursday......................................
Friday......................................
Saturday......................................

TOP GOALS

TOP TO DO OF THE WEEK

HEALTHY EATING TRACKER

M	T	W	T	F	S	S
☐	☐	☐	☐	☐	☐	☐
☐	☐	☐	☐	☐	☐	☐
☐	☐	☐	☐	☐	☐	☐
☐	☐	☐	☐	☐	☐	☐
☐	☐	☐	☐	☐	☐	☐
☐	☐	☐	☐	☐	☐	☐
☐	☐	☐	☐	☐	☐	☐
☐	☐	☐	☐	☐	☐	☐

QUOTE OF THE DAY

TODAY I AM GRATEFUL FOR:

My Week at a Glance

Week of: ____________________

MY WEEKLY AGENDA: NOTES

Sunday..

Monday..

Tuesday..

Wednesday..

Thursday..

Friday..

Saturday..

TOP GOALS

TOP TO DO OF THE WEEK

HEALTHY EATING TRACKER

M	T	W	T	F	S	S

QUOTE OF THE DAY

TODAY I AM GRATEFUL FOR:

My Week at a Glance

Week of: ____________________

MY WEEKLY AGENDA: NOTES

Sunday..

Monday..

Tuesday..

Wednesday..

Thursday..

Friday..

Saturday..

TOP GOALS

TOP TO DO OF THE WEEK

HEALTHY EATING TRACKER

M	T	W	T	F	S	S

QUOTE OF THE DAY

TODAY I AM GRATEFUL FOR:

My Week at a Glance

Week of:____________________

MY WEEKLY AGENDA: NOTES

Sunday..

Monday..

Tuesday..

Wednesday..

Thursday..

Friday..

Saturday..

TOP GOALS

TOP TO DO OF THE WEEK

HEALTHY EATING TRACKER

M	T	W	T	F	S	S

QUOTE OF THE DAY

TODAY I AM GRATEFUL FOR:

My Week at a Glance

Week of:____________________

MY WEEKLY AGENDA: NOTES

Sunday..

Monday..

Tuesday..

Wednesday..

Thursday..

Friday...

Saturday...

TOP GOALS

TOP TO DO OF THE WEEK

HEALTHY EATING TRACKER

M	T	W	T	F	S	S
☐	☐	☐	☐	☐	☐	☐
☐	☐	☐	☐	☐	☐	☐
☐	☐	☐	☐	☐	☐	☐
☐	☐	☐	☐	☐	☐	☐
☐	☐	☐	☐	☐	☐	☐
☐	☐	☐	☐	☐	☐	☐
☐	☐	☐	☐	☐	☐	☐
☐	☐	☐	☐	☐	☐	☐

QUOTE OF THE DAY

TODAY I AM GRATEFUL FOR:

My Week at a Glance

Week of: ____________________

MY WEEKLY AGENDA: NOTES

Sunday..

Monday..

Tuesday..

Wednesday..

Thursday..

Friday..

Saturday..

TOP GOALS

TOP TO DO OF THE WEEK

HEALTHY EATING TRACKER

M	T	W	T	F	S	S
☐	☐	☐	☐	☐	☐	☐
☐	☐	☐	☐	☐	☐	☐
☐	☐	☐	☐	☐	☐	☐
☐	☐	☐	☐	☐	☐	☐
☐	☐	☐	☐	☐	☐	☐
☐	☐	☐	☐	☐	☐	☐
☐	☐	☐	☐	☐	☐	☐
☐	☐	☐	☐	☐	☐	☐

QUOTE OF THE DAY

TODAY I AM GRATEFUL FOR:

My Week at a Glance

Week of: ____________________

MY WEEKLY AGENDA: NOTES

Sunday..

Monday..

Tuesday..

Wednesday..

Thursday..

Friday..

Saturday..

TOP GOALS

TOP TO DO OF THE WEEK

HEALTHY EATING TRACKER

M	T	W	T	F	S	S
☐	☐	☐	☐	☐	☐	☐
☐	☐	☐	☐	☐	☐	☐
☐	☐	☐	☐	☐	☐	☐
☐	☐	☐	☐	☐	☐	☐
☐	☐	☐	☐	☐	☐	☐
☐	☐	☐	☐	☐	☐	☐
☐	☐	☐	☐	☐	☐	☐
☐	☐	☐	☐	☐	☐	☐

QUOTE OF THE DAY

TODAY I AM GRATEFUL FOR:

My Week at a Glance

Week of: ____________________

MY WEEKLY AGENDA: NOTES

Sunday..

Monday..

Tuesday..

Wednesday..

Thursday..

Friday..

Saturday..

TOP GOALS

TOP TO DO OF THE WEEK

HEALTHY EATING TRACKER

M	T	W	T	F	S	S
☐	☐	☐	☐	☐	☐	☐
☐	☐	☐	☐	☐	☐	☐
☐	☐	☐	☐	☐	☐	☐
☐	☐	☐	☐	☐	☐	☐
☐	☐	☐	☐	☐	☐	☐
☐	☐	☐	☐	☐	☐	☐
☐	☐	☐	☐	☐	☐	☐
☐	☐	☐	☐	☐	☐	☐

QUOTE OF THE DAY

TODAY I AM GRATEFUL FOR:

My Week at a Glance

Week of: ____________________

MY WEEKLY AGENDA: NOTES

Sunday..

Monday..

Tuesday..

Wednesday..

Thursday..

Friday..

Saturday..

TOP GOALS

TOP TO DO OF THE WEEK

HEALTHY EATING TRACKER

M	T	W	T	F	S	S
☐	☐	☐	☐	☐	☐	☐
☐	☐	☐	☐	☐	☐	☐
☐	☐	☐	☐	☐	☐	☐
☐	☐	☐	☐	☐	☐	☐
☐	☐	☐	☐	☐	☐	☐
☐	☐	☐	☐	☐	☐	☐
☐	☐	☐	☐	☐	☐	☐
☐	☐	☐	☐	☐	☐	☐

QUOTE OF THE DAY

TODAY I AM GRATEFUL FOR:

My Week at a Glance

Week of: ____________________

MY WEEKLY AGENDA: NOTES

Sunday..

Monday..

Tuesday..

Wednesday..

Thursday..

Friday..

Saturday..

TOP GOALS

HEALTHY EATING TRACKER

M	T	W	T	F	S	S
☐	☐	☐	☐	☐	☐	☐
☐	☐	☐	☐	☐	☐	☐
☐	☐	☐	☐	☐	☐	☐
☐	☐	☐	☐	☐	☐	☐
☐	☐	☐	☐	☐	☐	☐
☐	☐	☐	☐	☐	☐	☐
☐	☐	☐	☐	☐	☐	☐
☐	☐	☐	☐	☐	☐	☐

TOP TO DO OF THE WEEK

QUOTE OF THE DAY

TODAY I AM GRATEFUL FOR:

My Week at a Glance

Week of: ____________________

MY WEEKLY AGENDA: NOTES

Sunday..

Monday..

Tuesday..

Wednesday..

Thursday..

Friday..

Saturday..

TOP GOALS

TOP TO DO OF THE WEEK

HEALTHY EATING TRACKER

M	T	W	T	F	S	S

QUOTE OF THE DAY

TODAY I AM GRATEFUL FOR:

My Week at a Glance

Week of: ____________________

MY WEEKLY AGENDA: NOTES

Sunday..........

Monday..........

Tuesday..........

Wednesday..........

Thursday..........

Friday..........

Saturday..........

TOP GOALS

TOP TO DO OF THE WEEK

HEALTHY EATING TRACKER

M	T	W	T	F	S	S

QUOTE OF THE DAY

TODAY I AM GRATEFUL FOR:

My Week at a Glance

Week of: ____________________

MY WEEKLY AGENDA: NOTES

Sunday..
Monday..
Tuesday..
Wednesday..
Thursday..
Friday..
Saturday..

TOP GOALS

HEALTHY EATING TRACKER

M	T	W	T	F	S	S
☐	☐	☐	☐	☐	☐	☐
☐	☐	☐	☐	☐	☐	☐
☐	☐	☐	☐	☐	☐	☐
☐	☐	☐	☐	☐	☐	☐
☐	☐	☐	☐	☐	☐	☐
☐	☐	☐	☐	☐	☐	☐
☐	☐	☐	☐	☐	☐	☐
☐	☐	☐	☐	☐	☐	☐

TOP TO DO OF THE WEEK

QUOTE OF THE DAY

TODAY I AM GRATEFUL FOR:

My Week at a Glance

Week of: ____________________

MY WEEKLY AGENDA: NOTES

Sunday..

Monday..

Tuesday..

Wednesday..

Thursday..

Friday..

Saturday..

TOP GOALS

HEALTHY EATING TRACKER

M	T	W	T	F	S	S
☐	☐	☐	☐	☐	☐	☐
☐	☐	☐	☐	☐	☐	☐
☐	☐	☐	☐	☐	☐	☐
☐	☐	☐	☐	☐	☐	☐
☐	☐	☐	☐	☐	☐	☐
☐	☐	☐	☐	☐	☐	☐
☐	☐	☐	☐	☐	☐	☐
☐	☐	☐	☐	☐	☐	☐

TOP TO DO OF THE WEEK

QUOTE OF THE DAY

TODAY I AM GRATEFUL FOR:

My Week at a Glance

Week of: ____________________

MY WEEKLY AGENDA: NOTES

Sunday..

Monday..

Tuesday..

Wednesday..

Thursday..

Friday..

Saturday..

TOP GOALS

TOP TO DO OF THE WEEK

HEALTHY EATING TRACKER

M	T	W	T	F	S	S
☐	☐	☐	☐	☐	☐	☐
☐	☐	☐	☐	☐	☐	☐
☐	☐	☐	☐	☐	☐	☐
☐	☐	☐	☐	☐	☐	☐
☐	☐	☐	☐	☐	☐	☐
☐	☐	☐	☐	☐	☐	☐
☐	☐	☐	☐	☐	☐	☐
☐	☐	☐	☐	☐	☐	☐

QUOTE OF THE DAY

TODAY I AM GRATEFUL FOR:

My Week at a Glance

Week of: ____________________

MY WEEKLY AGENDA: NOTES
Sunday
Monday
Tuesday
Wednesday
Thursday
Friday
Saturday

TOP GOALS

TOP TO DO OF THE WEEK

HEALTHY EATING TRACKER

M	T	W	T	F	S	S
☐	☐	☐	☐	☐	☐	☐
☐	☐	☐	☐	☐	☐	☐
☐	☐	☐	☐	☐	☐	☐
☐	☐	☐	☐	☐	☐	☐
☐	☐	☐	☐	☐	☐	☐
☐	☐	☐	☐	☐	☐	☐
☐	☐	☐	☐	☐	☐	☐
☐	☐	☐	☐	☐	☐	☐

QUOTE OF THE DAY

TODAY I AM GRATEFUL FOR:

My Week at a Glance

Week of: ____________________

MY WEEKLY AGENDA: NOTES

Sunday..

Monday..

Tuesday..

Wednesday..

Thursday..

Friday..

Saturday..

TOP GOALS

TOP TO DO OF THE WEEK

HEALTHY EATING TRACKER

M	T	W	T	F	S	S
☐	☐	☐	☐	☐	☐	☐
☐	☐	☐	☐	☐	☐	☐
☐	☐	☐	☐	☐	☐	☐
☐	☐	☐	☐	☐	☐	☐
☐	☐	☐	☐	☐	☐	☐
☐	☐	☐	☐	☐	☐	☐
☐	☐	☐	☐	☐	☐	☐
☐	☐	☐	☐	☐	☐	☐

QUOTE OF THE DAY

TODAY I AM GRATEFUL FOR:

My Week at a Glance

Week of: ____________________

MY WEEKLY AGENDA: NOTES

Sunday..

Monday..

Tuesday..

Wednesday..

Thursday..

Friday..

Saturday..

TOP GOALS

TOP TO DO OF THE WEEK

HEALTHY EATING TRACKER

M	T	W	T	F	S	S
☐	☐	☐	☐	☐	☐	☐
☐	☐	☐	☐	☐	☐	☐
☐	☐	☐	☐	☐	☐	☐
☐	☐	☐	☐	☐	☐	☐
☐	☐	☐	☐	☐	☐	☐
☐	☐	☐	☐	☐	☐	☐
☐	☐	☐	☐	☐	☐	☐
☐	☐	☐	☐	☐	☐	☐

QUOTE OF THE DAY

TODAY I AM GRATEFUL FOR:

My Week at a Glance

Week of: ____________________

MY WEEKLY AGENDA: NOTES

Sunday..

Monday..

Tuesday..

Wednesday..

Thursday..

Friday..

Saturday..

TOP GOALS

HEALTHY EATING TRACKER

M	T	W	T	F	S	S
☐	☐	☐	☐	☐	☐	☐
☐	☐	☐	☐	☐	☐	☐
☐	☐	☐	☐	☐	☐	☐
☐	☐	☐	☐	☐	☐	☐
☐	☐	☐	☐	☐	☐	☐
☐	☐	☐	☐	☐	☐	☐
☐	☐	☐	☐	☐	☐	☐
☐	☐	☐	☐	☐	☐	☐

TOP TO DO OF THE WEEK

QUOTE OF THE DAY

TODAY I AM GRATEFUL FOR:

My Week at a Glance

Week of: ____________________

MY WEEKLY AGENDA: NOTES

Sunday..........

Monday..........

Tuesday..........

Wednesday..........

Thursday..........

Friday..........

Saturday..........

TOP GOALS

TOP TO DO OF THE WEEK

HEALTHY EATING TRACKER

M	T	W	T	F	S	S

QUOTE OF THE DAY

TODAY I AM GRATEFUL FOR:

My Week at a Glance

Week of: ____________________

MY WEEKLY AGENDA: NOTES

Sunday..

Monday..

Tuesday..

Wednesday..

Thursday..

Friday..

Saturday..

TOP GOALS

TOP TO DO OF THE WEEK

HEALTHY EATING TRACKER

M	T	W	T	F	S	S
☐	☐	☐	☐	☐	☐	☐
☐	☐	☐	☐	☐	☐	☐
☐	☐	☐	☐	☐	☐	☐
☐	☐	☐	☐	☐	☐	☐
☐	☐	☐	☐	☐	☐	☐
☐	☐	☐	☐	☐	☐	☐
☐	☐	☐	☐	☐	☐	☐
☐	☐	☐	☐	☐	☐	☐

QUOTE OF THE DAY

TODAY I AM GRATEFUL FOR:

My Week at a Glance

Week of: ____________________

MY WEEKLY AGENDA: NOTES

Sunday..

Monday..

Tuesday..

Wednesday..

Thursday..

Friday..

Saturday..

TOP GOALS

HEALTHY EATING TRACKER

M	T	W	T	F	S	S
☐	☐	☐	☐	☐	☐	☐
☐	☐	☐	☐	☐	☐	☐
☐	☐	☐	☐	☐	☐	☐
☐	☐	☐	☐	☐	☐	☐
☐	☐	☐	☐	☐	☐	☐
☐	☐	☐	☐	☐	☐	☐
☐	☐	☐	☐	☐	☐	☐
☐	☐	☐	☐	☐	☐	☐

TOP TO DO OF THE WEEK

QUOTE OF THE DAY

TODAY I AM GRATEFUL FOR:

My Week at a Glance

Week of: ____________________

MY WEEKLY AGENDA: NOTES

Sunday..

Monday..

Tuesday..

Wednesday..

Thursday..

Friday..

Saturday..

TOP GOALS

TOP TO DO OF THE WEEK

HEALTHY EATING TRACKER

M	T	W	T	F	S	S
☐	☐	☐	☐	☐	☐	☐
☐	☐	☐	☐	☐	☐	☐
☐	☐	☐	☐	☐	☐	☐
☐	☐	☐	☐	☐	☐	☐
☐	☐	☐	☐	☐	☐	☐
☐	☐	☐	☐	☐	☐	☐
☐	☐	☐	☐	☐	☐	☐
☐	☐	☐	☐	☐	☐	☐

QUOTE OF THE DAY

TODAY I AM GRATEFUL FOR:

My Week at a Glance

Week of: ____________________

MY WEEKLY AGENDA: NOTES

Sunday..

Monday..

Tuesday..

Wednesday..

Thursday..

Friday..

Saturday..

TOP GOALS

TOP TO DO OF THE WEEK

HEALTHY EATING TRACKER

M	T	W	T	F	S	S

QUOTE OF THE DAY

TODAY I AM GRATEFUL FOR:

My Week at a Glance

Week of: ____________________

MY WEEKLY AGENDA: NOTES

Sunday..

Monday..

Tuesday..

Wednesday..

Thursday..

Friday..

Saturday..

TOP GOALS

TOP TO DO OF THE WEEK

HEALTHY EATING TRACKER

M	T	W	T	F	S	S
☐	☐	☐	☐	☐	☐	☐
☐	☐	☐	☐	☐	☐	☐
☐	☐	☐	☐	☐	☐	☐
☐	☐	☐	☐	☐	☐	☐
☐	☐	☐	☐	☐	☐	☐
☐	☐	☐	☐	☐	☐	☐
☐	☐	☐	☐	☐	☐	☐
☐	☐	☐	☐	☐	☐	☐

QUOTE OF THE DAY

TODAY I AM GRATEFUL FOR:

My Week at a Glance

Week of:__________________

MY WEEKLY AGENDA: NOTES

Sunday..........

Monday..........

Tuesday..........

Wednesday..........

Thursday..........

Friday..........

Saturday..........

TOP GOALS

TOP TO DO OF THE WEEK

HEALTHY EATING TRACKER

M	T	W	T	F	S	S
☐	☐	☐	☐	☐	☐	☐
☐	☐	☐	☐	☐	☐	☐
☐	☐	☐	☐	☐	☐	☐
☐	☐	☐	☐	☐	☐	☐
☐	☐	☐	☐	☐	☐	☐
☐	☐	☐	☐	☐	☐	☐
☐	☐	☐	☐	☐	☐	☐
☐	☐	☐	☐	☐	☐	☐

QUOTE OF THE DAY

TODAY I AM GRATEFUL FOR:

My Week at a Glance

Week of: ____________________

MY WEEKLY AGENDA: NOTES

Sunday..

Monday..

Tuesday..

Wednesday..

Thursday..

Friday..

Saturday..

TOP GOALS

TOP TO DO OF THE WEEK

HEALTHY EATING TRACKER

M	T	W	T	F	S	S
☐	☐	☐	☐	☐	☐	☐
☐	☐	☐	☐	☐	☐	☐
☐	☐	☐	☐	☐	☐	☐
☐	☐	☐	☐	☐	☐	☐
☐	☐	☐	☐	☐	☐	☐
☐	☐	☐	☐	☐	☐	☐
☐	☐	☐	☐	☐	☐	☐
☐	☐	☐	☐	☐	☐	☐

QUOTE OF THE DAY

TODAY I AM GRATEFUL FOR:

My Week at a Glance

Week of: ____________________

MY WEEKLY AGENDA: NOTES

Sunday..

Monday..

Tuesday..

Wednesday..

Thursday..

Friday..

Saturday..

TOP GOALS

HEALTHY EATING TRACKER

M	T	W	T	F	S	S
☐	☐	☐	☐	☐	☐	☐
☐	☐	☐	☐	☐	☐	☐
☐	☐	☐	☐	☐	☐	☐
☐	☐	☐	☐	☐	☐	☐
☐	☐	☐	☐	☐	☐	☐
☐	☐	☐	☐	☐	☐	☐
☐	☐	☐	☐	☐	☐	☐
☐	☐	☐	☐	☐	☐	☐

TOP TO DO OF THE WEEK

☐ ____________________

☐ ____________________

☐ ____________________

☐ ____________________

QUOTE OF THE DAY

TODAY I AM GRATEFUL FOR:

My Week at a Glance

Week of: ______________________

MY WEEKLY AGENDA: NOTES

Sunday..

Monday..

Tuesday..

Wednesday..

Thursday..

Friday..

Saturday..

TOP GOALS

TOP TO DO OF THE WEEK

HEALTHY EATING TRACKER

M	T	W	T	F	S	S
☐	☐	☐	☐	☐	☐	☐
☐	☐	☐	☐	☐	☐	☐
☐	☐	☐	☐	☐	☐	☐
☐	☐	☐	☐	☐	☐	☐
☐	☐	☐	☐	☐	☐	☐
☐	☐	☐	☐	☐	☐	☐
☐	☐	☐	☐	☐	☐	☐
☐	☐	☐	☐	☐	☐	☐

QUOTE OF THE DAY

TODAY I AM GRATEFUL FOR:

My Week at a Glance

Week of: ____________________

MY WEEKLY AGENDA: NOTES

Sunday..

Monday..

Tuesday..

Wednesday..

Thursday..

Friday..

Saturday..

TOP GOALS

HEALTHY EATING TRACKER

M	T	W	T	F	S	S
☐	☐	☐	☐	☐	☐	☐
☐	☐	☐	☐	☐	☐	☐
☐	☐	☐	☐	☐	☐	☐
☐	☐	☐	☐	☐	☐	☐
☐	☐	☐	☐	☐	☐	☐
☐	☐	☐	☐	☐	☐	☐
☐	☐	☐	☐	☐	☐	☐
☐	☐	☐	☐	☐	☐	☐

TOP TO DO OF THE WEEK

QUOTE OF THE DAY

TODAY I AM GRATEFUL FOR:

My Week at a Glance

Week of: ____________

MY WEEKLY AGENDA: NOTES

Sunday..

Monday..

Tuesday..

Wednesday..

Thursday..

Friday..

Saturday..

TOP GOALS

HEALTHY EATING TRACKER

M	T	W	T	F	S	S
☐	☐	☐	☐	☐	☐	☐
☐	☐	☐	☐	☐	☐	☐
☐	☐	☐	☐	☐	☐	☐
☐	☐	☐	☐	☐	☐	☐
☐	☐	☐	☐	☐	☐	☐
☐	☐	☐	☐	☐	☐	☐
☐	☐	☐	☐	☐	☐	☐
☐	☐	☐	☐	☐	☐	☐

TOP TO DO OF THE WEEK

QUOTE OF THE DAY

TODAY I AM GRATEFUL FOR:

My Week at a Glance

Week of: ____________________

MY WEEKLY AGENDA: NOTES

Sunday..

Monday..

Tuesday..

Wednesday..

Thursday..

Friday..

Saturday..

TOP GOALS

HEALTHY EATING TRACKER

M	T	W	T	F	S	S
☐	☐	☐	☐	☐	☐	☐
☐	☐	☐	☐	☐	☐	☐
☐	☐	☐	☐	☐	☐	☐
☐	☐	☐	☐	☐	☐	☐
☐	☐	☐	☐	☐	☐	☐
☐	☐	☐	☐	☐	☐	☐
☐	☐	☐	☐	☐	☐	☐
☐	☐	☐	☐	☐	☐	☐

TOP TO DO OF THE WEEK

☐ ____________________

☐ ____________________

☐ ____________________

☐ ____________________

QUOTE OF THE DAY

TODAY I AM GRATEFUL FOR:

My Week at a Glance

Week of: ____________________

MY WEEKLY AGENDA: NOTES

Sunday..

Monday..

Tuesday..

Wednesday..

Thursday..

Friday..

Saturday..

TOP GOALS

TOP TO DO OF THE WEEK

HEALTHY EATING TRACKER

M	T	W	T	F	S	S

QUOTE OF THE DAY

TODAY I AM GRATEFUL FOR:

My Week at a Glance

Week of: ____________________

MY WEEKLY AGENDA: NOTES

Sunday..

Monday..

Tuesday..

Wednesday..

Thursday..

Friday..

Saturday..

TOP GOALS

TOP TO DO OF THE WEEK

HEALTHY EATING TRACKER

M	T	W	T	F	S	S
☐	☐	☐	☐	☐	☐	☐
☐	☐	☐	☐	☐	☐	☐
☐	☐	☐	☐	☐	☐	☐
☐	☐	☐	☐	☐	☐	☐
☐	☐	☐	☐	☐	☐	☐
☐	☐	☐	☐	☐	☐	☐
☐	☐	☐	☐	☐	☐	☐
☐	☐	☐	☐	☐	☐	☐

QUOTE OF THE DAY

TODAY I AM GRATEFUL FOR:

My Week at a Glance

Week of: ____________________

MY WEEKLY AGENDA: NOTES

Sunday..

Monday..

Tuesday..

Wednesday..

Thursday..

Friday..

Saturday..

TOP GOALS

HEALTHY EATING TRACKER

M	T	W	T	F	S	S
☐	☐	☐	☐	☐	☐	☐
☐	☐	☐	☐	☐	☐	☐
☐	☐	☐	☐	☐	☐	☐
☐	☐	☐	☐	☐	☐	☐
☐	☐	☐	☐	☐	☐	☐
☐	☐	☐	☐	☐	☐	☐
☐	☐	☐	☐	☐	☐	☐
☐	☐	☐	☐	☐	☐	☐

TOP TO DO OF THE WEEK

☐ ____________________

☐ ____________________

☐ ____________________

☐ ____________________

QUOTE OF THE DAY

TODAY I AM GRATEFUL FOR:

My Week at a Glance

Week of: ____________________

MY WEEKLY AGENDA: NOTES

Sunday……………………………………

Monday……………………………………

Tuesday……………………………………

Wednesday……………………………………

Thursday……………………………………

Friday……………………………………

Saturday……………………………………

TOP GOALS

TOP TO DO OF THE WEEK

HEALTHY EATING TRACKER

M	T	W	T	F	S	S
☐	☐	☐	☐	☐	☐	☐
☐	☐	☐	☐	☐	☐	☐
☐	☐	☐	☐	☐	☐	☐
☐	☐	☐	☐	☐	☐	☐
☐	☐	☐	☐	☐	☐	☐
☐	☐	☐	☐	☐	☐	☐
☐	☐	☐	☐	☐	☐	☐
☐	☐	☐	☐	☐	☐	☐

QUOTE OF THE DAY

TODAY I AM GRATEFUL FOR:

My Week at a Glance

Week of: ____________________

MY WEEKLY AGENDA: NOTES

Sunday..........

Monday..........

Tuesday..........

Wednesday..........

Thursday..........

Friday..........

Saturday..........

TOP GOALS

TOP TO DO OF THE WEEK

HEALTHY EATING TRACKER

M	T	W	T	F	S	S
☐	☐	☐	☐	☐	☐	☐
☐	☐	☐	☐	☐	☐	☐
☐	☐	☐	☐	☐	☐	☐
☐	☐	☐	☐	☐	☐	☐
☐	☐	☐	☐	☐	☐	☐
☐	☐	☐	☐	☐	☐	☐
☐	☐	☐	☐	☐	☐	☐
☐	☐	☐	☐	☐	☐	☐

QUOTE OF THE DAY

TODAY I AM GRATEFUL FOR:

My Week at a Glance

Week of:__________________

MY WEEKLY AGENDA: NOTES

Sunday..

Monday..

Tuesday..

Wednesday..

Thursday..

Friday..

Saturday..

TOP GOALS

TOP TO DO OF THE WEEK

HEALTHY EATING TRACKER

M	T	W	T	F	S	S
☐	☐	☐	☐	☐	☐	☐
☐	☐	☐	☐	☐	☐	☐
☐	☐	☐	☐	☐	☐	☐
☐	☐	☐	☐	☐	☐	☐
☐	☐	☐	☐	☐	☐	☐
☐	☐	☐	☐	☐	☐	☐
☐	☐	☐	☐	☐	☐	☐
☐	☐	☐	☐	☐	☐	☐

QUOTE OF THE DAY

TODAY I AM GRATEFUL FOR:

My Week at a Glance

Week of: ____________________

MY WEEKLY AGENDA: NOTES

Sunday..

Monday..

Tuesday..

Wednesday..

Thursday..

Friday..

Saturday..

TOP GOALS

TOP TO DO OF THE WEEK

HEALTHY EATING TRACKER

M	T	W	T	F	S	S
☐	☐	☐	☐	☐	☐	☐
☐	☐	☐	☐	☐	☐	☐
☐	☐	☐	☐	☐	☐	☐
☐	☐	☐	☐	☐	☐	☐
☐	☐	☐	☐	☐	☐	☐
☐	☐	☐	☐	☐	☐	☐
☐	☐	☐	☐	☐	☐	☐
☐	☐	☐	☐	☐	☐	☐

QUOTE OF THE DAY

TODAY I AM GRATEFUL FOR:

My Week at a Glance

Week of: ____________________

MY WEEKLY AGENDA: NOTES

Sunday..

Monday..

Tuesday..

Wednesday..

Thursday..

Friday..

Saturday..

TOP GOALS

HEALTHY EATING TRACKER

M	T	W	T	F	S	S
☐	☐	☐	☐	☐	☐	☐
☐	☐	☐	☐	☐	☐	☐
☐	☐	☐	☐	☐	☐	☐
☐	☐	☐	☐	☐	☐	☐
☐	☐	☐	☐	☐	☐	☐
☐	☐	☐	☐	☐	☐	☐
☐	☐	☐	☐	☐	☐	☐
☐	☐	☐	☐	☐	☐	☐

TOP TO DO OF THE WEEK

☐ ____________________

☐ ____________________

☐ ____________________

☐ ____________________

QUOTE OF THE DAY

TODAY I AM GRATEFUL FOR:

My Week at a Glance

Week of: ____________________

MY WEEKLY AGENDA: NOTES

Sunday..

Monday..

Tuesday..

Wednesday..

Thursday..

Friday..

Saturday..

TOP GOALS

TOP TO DO OF THE WEEK

HEALTHY EATING TRACKER

M	T	W	T	F	S	S
☐	☐	☐	☐	☐	☐	☐
☐	☐	☐	☐	☐	☐	☐
☐	☐	☐	☐	☐	☐	☐
☐	☐	☐	☐	☐	☐	☐
☐	☐	☐	☐	☐	☐	☐
☐	☐	☐	☐	☐	☐	☐
☐	☐	☐	☐	☐	☐	☐
☐	☐	☐	☐	☐	☐	☐

QUOTE OF THE DAY

TODAY I AM GRATEFUL FOR:

My Week at a Glance

Week of: ____________________

MY WEEKLY AGENDA: NOTES

Sunday..

Monday..

Tuesday..

Wednesday..

Thursday..

Friday..

Saturday..

TOP GOALS

TOP TO DO OF THE WEEK

HEALTHY EATING TRACKER

M	T	W	T	F	S	S
☐	☐	☐	☐	☐	☐	☐
☐	☐	☐	☐	☐	☐	☐
☐	☐	☐	☐	☐	☐	☐
☐	☐	☐	☐	☐	☐	☐
☐	☐	☐	☐	☐	☐	☐
☐	☐	☐	☐	☐	☐	☐
☐	☐	☐	☐	☐	☐	☐
☐	☐	☐	☐	☐	☐	☐

QUOTE OF THE DAY

TODAY I AM GRATEFUL FOR:

My Week at a Glance

Week of: ____________________

MY WEEKLY AGENDA: NOTES

Sunday..

Monday..

Tuesday..

Wednesday..

Thursday..

Friday..

Saturday..

TOP GOALS

TOP TO DO OF THE WEEK

HEALTHY EATING TRACKER

M	T	W	T	F	S	S
☐	☐	☐	☐	☐	☐	☐
☐	☐	☐	☐	☐	☐	☐
☐	☐	☐	☐	☐	☐	☐
☐	☐	☐	☐	☐	☐	☐
☐	☐	☐	☐	☐	☐	☐
☐	☐	☐	☐	☐	☐	☐
☐	☐	☐	☐	☐	☐	☐
☐	☐	☐	☐	☐	☐	☐

QUOTE OF THE DAY

TODAY I AM GRATEFUL FOR:

My Week at a Glance

Week of: ____________________

MY WEEKLY AGENDA: NOTES

Sunday..

Monday..

Tuesday..

Wednesday..

Thursday..

Friday..

Saturday..

TOP GOALS

TOP TO DO OF THE WEEK

HEALTHY EATING TRACKER

M	T	W	T	F	S	S
☐	☐	☐	☐	☐	☐	☐
☐	☐	☐	☐	☐	☐	☐
☐	☐	☐	☐	☐	☐	☐
☐	☐	☐	☐	☐	☐	☐
☐	☐	☐	☐	☐	☐	☐
☐	☐	☐	☐	☐	☐	☐
☐	☐	☐	☐	☐	☐	☐
☐	☐	☐	☐	☐	☐	☐

QUOTE OF THE DAY

TODAY I AM GRATEFUL FOR:

My Week at a Glance

Week of: ____________________

MY WEEKLY AGENDA: NOTES

Sunday..

Monday..

Tuesday..

Wednesday..

Thursday..

Friday..

Saturday..

TOP GOALS

HEALTHY EATING TRACKER

M	T	W	T	F	S	S
☐	☐	☐	☐	☐	☐	☐
☐	☐	☐	☐	☐	☐	☐
☐	☐	☐	☐	☐	☐	☐
☐	☐	☐	☐	☐	☐	☐
☐	☐	☐	☐	☐	☐	☐
☐	☐	☐	☐	☐	☐	☐
☐	☐	☐	☐	☐	☐	☐
☐	☐	☐	☐	☐	☐	☐

TOP TO DO OF THE WEEK

☐ ____________________

☐ ____________________

☐ ____________________

☐ ____________________

QUOTE OF THE DAY

TODAY I AM GRATEFUL FOR:

My Week at a Glance

Week of:_______________________

MY WEEKLY AGENDA: NOTES

Sunday..

Monday..

Tuesday..

Wednesday..

Thursday..

Friday..

Saturday..

TOP GOALS

TOP TO DO OF THE WEEK

HEALTHY EATING TRACKER

M	T	W	T	F	S	S
☐	☐	☐	☐	☐	☐	☐
☐	☐	☐	☐	☐	☐	☐
☐	☐	☐	☐	☐	☐	☐
☐	☐	☐	☐	☐	☐	☐
☐	☐	☐	☐	☐	☐	☐
☐	☐	☐	☐	☐	☐	☐
☐	☐	☐	☐	☐	☐	☐
☐	☐	☐	☐	☐	☐	☐

QUOTE OF THE DAY

TODAY I AM GRATEFUL FOR:

My Week at a Glance

Week of: ____________________

MY WEEKLY AGENDA: NOTES

Sunday..

Monday..

Tuesday..

Wednesday..

Thursday..

Friday..

Saturday..

TOP GOALS

TOP TO DO OF THE WEEK

HEALTHY EATING TRACKER

M	T	W	T	F	S	S
☐	☐	☐	☐	☐	☐	☐
☐	☐	☐	☐	☐	☐	☐
☐	☐	☐	☐	☐	☐	☐
☐	☐	☐	☐	☐	☐	☐
☐	☐	☐	☐	☐	☐	☐
☐	☐	☐	☐	☐	☐	☐
☐	☐	☐	☐	☐	☐	☐
☐	☐	☐	☐	☐	☐	☐

QUOTE OF THE DAY

TODAY I AM GRATEFUL FOR:

Notes and Things

Coloring Pages

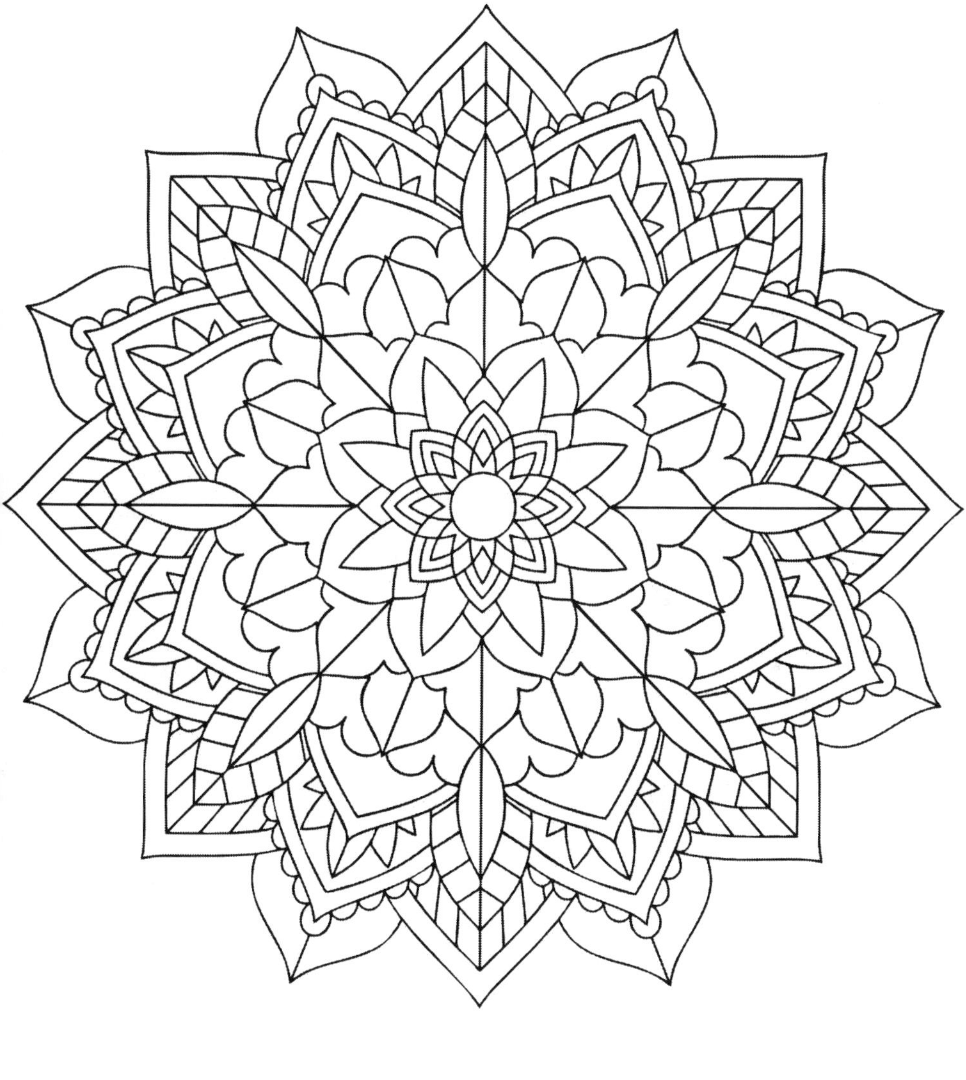

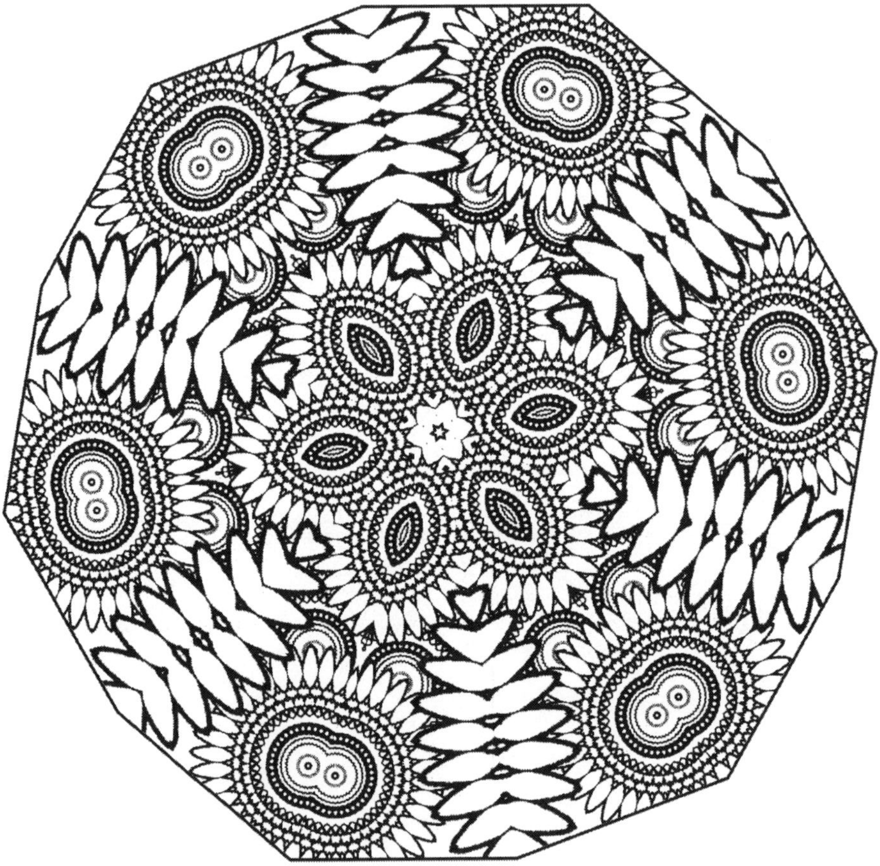

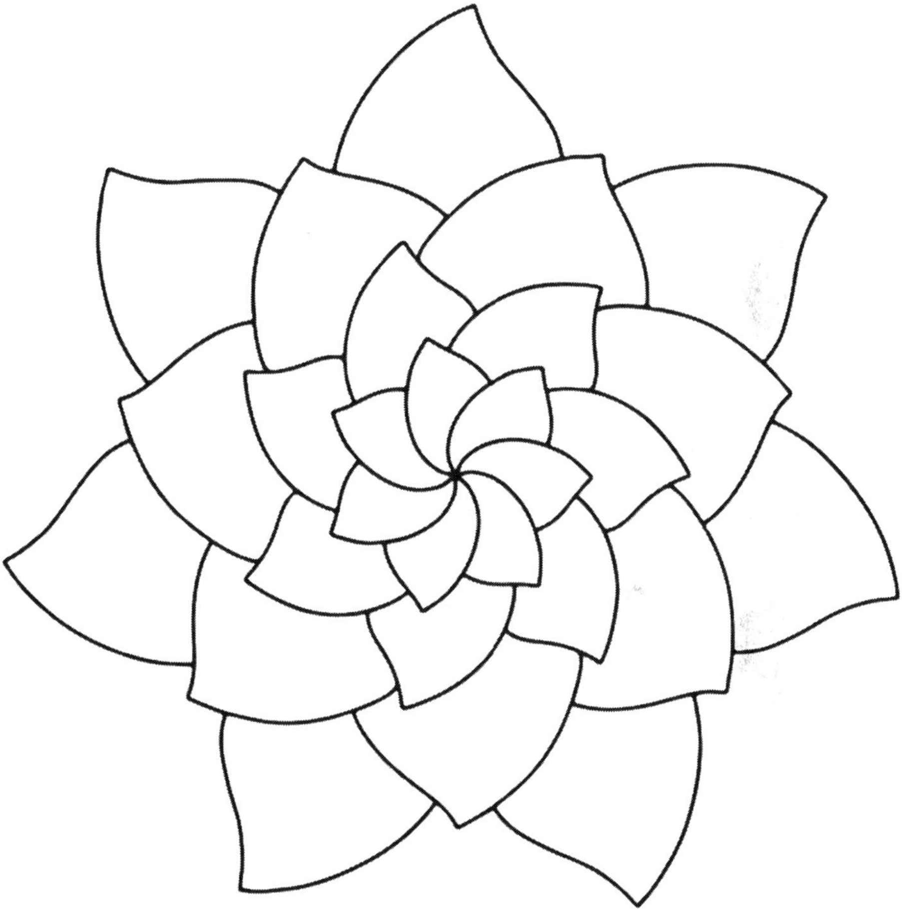

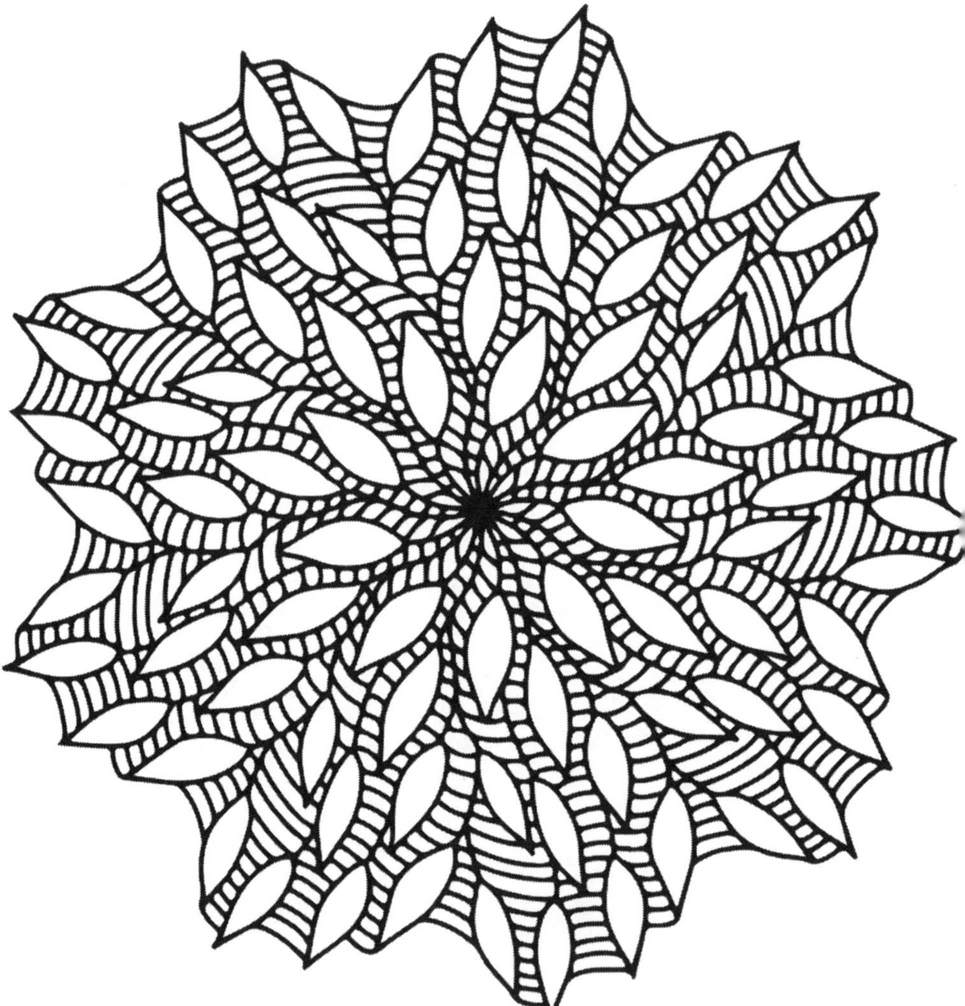

Made in the USA
Middletown, DE
02 October 2020

20994780R00052